How to Meditate

& Focus

for Success

in 10 Minutes a Day

Challenge Yourself & get Results

by

Louisa Marsh & Susie Ellis

"If the mind is the cause of all
our miseries, then surely the
same mind is the answer
to all our problems…

Stop looking elsewhere for
solutions, simply go within
& everything you need will
be there"

Sanjib Mukherjee 20 ii 2019

Table of Contents

Introduction

Meditation is one easy way to combat the effects of daily stress, and take back control of your health. Just 10 minutes a day can reduce stress and help your brain to recharge.

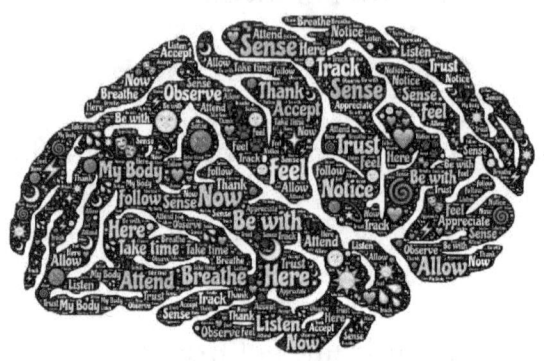

Today's world is always changing & people are starting to incorporate holistic mindful practices into their daily lives.

We probably all know someone who practices meditation. For some, it's a daily practice, while for others it's just for crisis situations. Crises are those moments where you feel as if your life is spinning out of control & moments when you just can't seem to get out of your own way.

Could you practice meditation? Maybe it appears too time consuming and not worth the trouble. If you think this way, you'll be in for an extremely pleasant surprise. Not only is meditation most certainly worth the time and effort, but the rewards speak for themselves.

There are many benefits associated with the practice of meditation which might surprise you. This book is going to help you to the heart of the subject & find out what meditation really is.

Meditation is available for everyone, you don't have to be a highly spiritual person or an expert in meditation with a certification to your name. It has a multitude of benefits.

CHAPTER 1: What is Meditation?

The art and practice of meditation basically has one goal in mind – to slow down the mind.

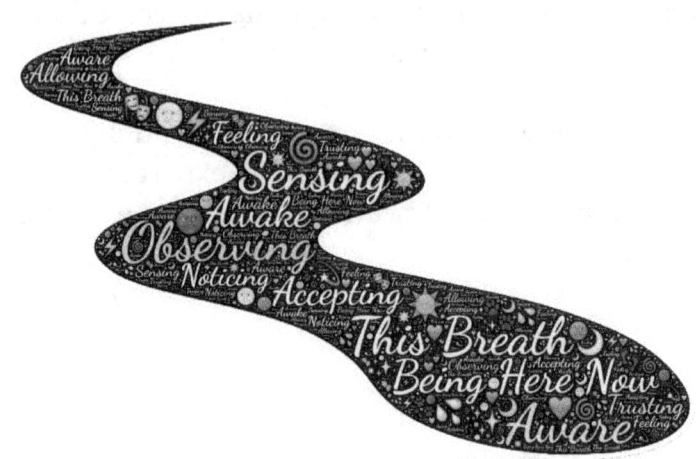

In today's culture, we all have such busy lifestyles and even busier minds, especially with our continued relationship with our phones on social media and the internet. Stress levels are up, blood pressure is up and relaxation is down. This is where meditation comes into play.

The practice of meditation has been around for centuries. People have used it for religious purposes and cultural reasons, however it now has credence in our secular society.

It isn't about becoming a new or different person, it's more about gaining a healthy sense of perspective, and training yourself in a sense of awareness, you are able to develop and have a different perspective, and observe the thoughts and feelings without always reacting to them!

The art and practice of meditation is one where you allow yourself and, most importantly to observe the mind without judgement and experience present-moment living. After all, if you really allow yourself to be present in any moment, without thought of what happened in the past or what is going to happen in the future, what a great sense of freedom and space this would give you.

Meditation takes time to master, after all you are learning to practice a new skill, that will allow you to relax, rest and rejuvenate yourself.

Initially your mind will wander off in all directions, this is perfectly normal, it's the human condition!

There are as many forms of meditation as there are practices, however we will introduce you to a simple 10 minute breathing meditation that will support you to make it a daily habit.

Through the art of breathing, learning to slow down your mind you come back to your centre which is the place within you where your deepest desires live and breathe, by sitting still you open yourself up to listening and feelings of peace. It's the place where you can move forward from and get back to and keep yourself on track.

The beauty of meditation is that it is available for everybody and will support you to have more focus and clarity in all areas of your life and from that place within creativity will flow.

Scientific research in this area has shown that the structure of the brainwaves can change. Meditation truly does have the power to change your mind(set) and allow you to think clearly. When you "shut" your mind up your subconscious mind, your deeper mind is given the space for limitless universal intelligence to come through and it's not so much the action of sitting down to meditate, it's the beginning of the action for your intention for a focused and successful life. It's an inside out job!

Chapter 2: The Power of Meditation

When we constantly replay in our mind all our worries, stress & anxieties, we affect our mental & physical health. What we focus on becomes a reality.

There is power in the way we control our attention as we meditate & begin to feel more relaxed and at peace. This peacefulness usually lasts far beyond the meditation itself.

Meditation teaches us how to respond, rather than react, to situations in our lives. It allows us to become more awake and more purposeful in our actions.

Meditation sounds simple, but it takes discipline to remain still in body and mind. We have to learn to block out the world around us and quieten our thoughts. To get the greatest benefit from meditation it is necessary to create a regular practice.

Some healthcare providers include meditation as part of their treatment for many conditions…

Among some of the benefits of meditation are:

- Lower blood pressure
- Decreased pain
- Improved function of the immune system
- Improved mood and brain function

You can read more about the benefits in Chapter 3.

Meditation can be broadly grouped into categories:

- Mindfulness ~ This focuses in on your thoughts and images as they appear.
- Concentrative ~ This focuses on your breathing, by repeating a certain phrase or sound, or by thinking about particular images.
- Transcendental ~ This develops the balance of your physical, mental, emotional & spiritual selves.
- Moving ~ This is a form of exercise that combines fitness with meditation.

There is power in meditation…

There are a number of theories on meditation which might improve our physical and mental health. One theory is that it reduces activity of the nervous system. This leads to a slower heart rate, lower blood pressure, slower breathing, and muscle relaxation.

There are several parts of the brain which are positively impacted by meditation:

- Frontal lobe
- Parietal lobe
- Thalamus

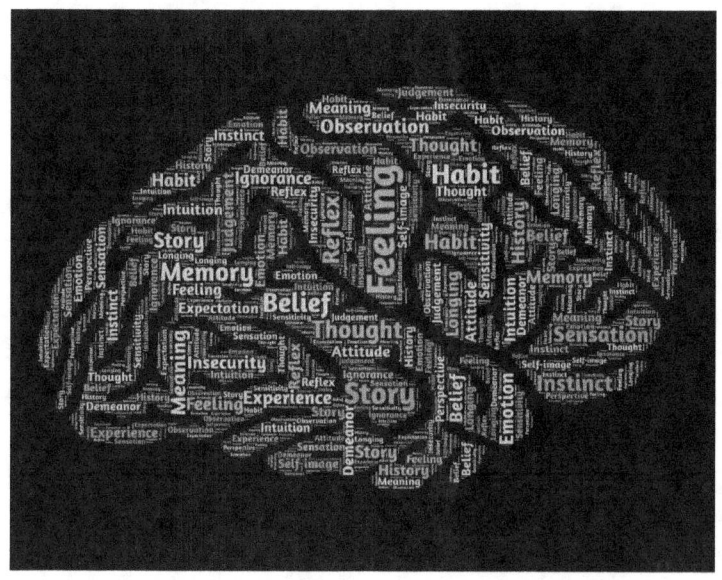

When we meditate our brainwaves
change. Meditation actually has the power to change
your mind & your mindset.

Using breathing techniques for example, our brain
waves have the capacity to slow down ~ the level of
beta waves in the brain are reduced. When the beta
waves slow down, we gain an overall sense of calm
and well-being.

Meditation affects the brain and the brain waves.
Each part of the brain, according to scientific studies
and research, is affected by meditation. Incoming
information can be slowed down when meditating so
that:

- Emotions are not as strong, they become diminished & not as volatile

- Sensory input slows down

- Worry, anxiety & over-thinking ceases to be impactful

- Mind chatter [the parrot on your shoulder] & information overload slows down

- We become connected to our inner powers of clarity, vitality & love

- It gives us an expanded sense of connection with all life & becomes an experience of profound joy

CHAPTER 3: The Benefits of Meditation

Why do so many people use and promote meditation? The answer is because it works. Meditation is successful for many reasons.

Here are 23 benefits… maybe you can think of more :)

1 Meditation Reduces Stress.

When you become stressed your body reacts with a fight or flight sensation… you either feel the need to take flight and run away to protect yourself or you feel the need to stay and fight. These bodily responses are natural but require peace to promote healing.

2 Meditation Decreases Anxiety

Some people have too much fight or flight syndrome & their gut instincts tell them they are in danger when they are really not. Meditation can help ease this anxiety.

The neural pathways in our brains need to determine whether or not we are in real, imminent danger. Sometimes these connections are so strong we feel we are in danger when we are not.

Meditation has a calming effect on our brain...reasoning is strengthened & irrational fears are weakened.

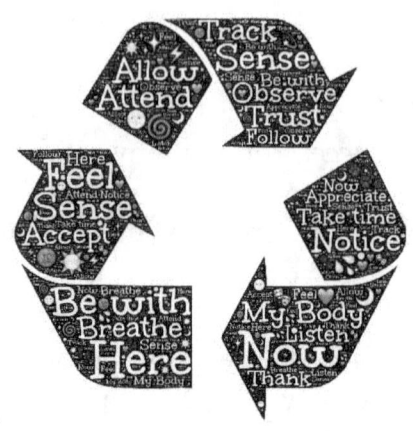

3 Meditation Promotes Emotional Health

Emotions can get out of control in all sorts of situations. Taking time out to meditate & re-think a dilemma has an immediate calming effect.

4 Meditation Enhances Self-Awareness

In our normal busy lives, we rarely take time out to consider ourselves, our inner being, our thought processes. Making space for a few minutes of meditation heightens our self-awareness & gives us insights that otherwise go unnoticed.

5 Meditation Lengthens Attention Span

Meditation has the power to re-align our thought processes. During this quiet time, we could choose to concentrate on a particular project or problem ~ give it a try, you might just be amazed.

6 Meditation May Reduce Age-Related Memory Loss

Our bodies & brains become tired as we age. We need to exercise our brains as well as our bodies. [Here is a great article on the subject] [1]

7 Meditation Can Generate Kindness

The most researched Buddhist kindness-based contemplative practice is the Loving-Kindness Meditation. The practice of loving-kindness is generated firstly for oneself to remove negative emotions that might impede our generating loving-kindness for others. There are some more interesting findings to read. [2]

8 Meditation May Help Fight Addictions.

A prominent 2005 study by Harvard neuroscientist Dr. Sara Lazar showed that meditators had significantly more neural density, cortical thickness, and overall activity within their prefrontal cortexes. Meditation will stimulate your brain to be happy & "naturally high", without the need for alcohol, prescriptions, marijuana, drugs, cigarettes, or any other addictive substance.

9 Meditation Enhances relationships

& allows you to become more emphatic. The neural pathways responsible for showing more compassion are activated. Scientific studies show that compassion and empathy are more active in someone who meditates.

10 Meditation & Children

"We need to help children find natural ways for body and mind to combat the pressures of modern living and to find better ways to help focus their minds on matters of importance. There are strong pedagogical reasons for including meditation as part of the daily experience of pupils of all ages and abilities". [3]

11 Meditation Improves memory & concentration

Meditation improves memory recall as it decreases distractions.

12. Meditation Eliminate mind chatter

The monkey mind, the parrot on your shoulder, or mind chatter can totally disable people. This is an exhausting but very common phenomenon. Buddha called this "kapicitta" & learned to drown it all out by slowing down the brain.

13 Meditation Increase Focus

Meditation can be used to declutter the mind. When we meditate, we are focused on the present moment & constant practice trains our brain...

14 Meditation Decreases Panic Attacks

The remedy of breathing into a paper bag is actually just focusing on breathing. By letting uncomfortable thoughts pass without reacting, you can develop a new response to fear and anxiety. Meditation & mindfulness allows you to detach from negative thinking by facing thoughts without reacting to them.

15 Meditation Unlocks Creativity

Meditation has a way of unlocking and unleashing creative potential. Over time, & with practice, mindfulness meditation can help create inner harmony, clarity, and peace. Unlocking creativity negates being stuck or experiencing writer's block for instance.

16 Meditation Enables "Nothingness"

Nothingness [śūnyatā or suññatā – pronounced 'shoonyataa'], is a concept which refers to a meditative state or experience. It is a way of clearing the mind making way for positive & creative thoughts.

17 Meditation Improves Sleep

We are all aware of the benefits of a good night's rest

- When you are well-rested, you are more productive
- When you get a good night's sleep, you are more focused
- When you are more focused, you are more successful

Meditation can help improve the quality of your sleep and make it easier to fall asleep and stay asleep.

Hundreds of thousands of people take medication to help them in get a decent night's sleep. These people suffer greatly from insomnia & no matter what they do they seem to keep tossing and turning.

They wake up in the morning feeling groggy and irritated, & they then get rundown or even sick.

Incorporating meditation into your nightly routine can help attain a more restful sleep. Deep breathing, concentrating on relaxing each part of your body in turn & repeating affirmations can all help.

18 Meditation Reduces Conflict

To gain a more compassionate approach to any conflict, meditation works through allowing us to move toward empathy and understanding. ... When we experience conflict emotions, we can meditate on compassion for ourselves & others & ease our mind away from anger or negativity.

19 Meditation & Establishing Our Own Boundaries

Do you find it hard to say 'no'? Are you wracked with guilt if you say 'no'? Meditation can help you establish what feels good for you. "Listen to your body to find your natural limits and healthy boundaries—along with core power, strength, and inner peace". [Bo Forbes PsyD 13/6/16]

20 Meditation, Happiness & Good Moods!

Meditation can make you smile more. People who meditate are shown to be more positive and upbeat. Meditation calms & soothes the mind. When the mind is calm, your spirit follows. Read an article by Forbes on the subject. [4]

21 Meditation & Self Love

It's easy to get lost in negative thoughts and self-doubt. Feelings of lack and insecurity make us feel worthy of love. Society condition us to believe that we must always be better i.e. thinner, happier, richer, smarter. Meditation can help us recognise that we are enough just as we are. Learn to love & appreciate who you are.

22 Meditation Can Slow Down the Ageing Process

A study published in 2013 [5] found that just 15 minutes' meditation in novices had immediate effects on the expression of many genes, for example increasing the activity of the gene that makes telomerase and reducing the activity of genes involved in inflammatory and stress responses. It's amazing what sitting still with your eyes closed and focusing on your breath can do for your cells. Here is a great article to read in the Guardian. [6]

23 Meditation Increases Brain Function

Meditation is exercise for your brain. The more you exercise your brain, the more you use it, the better it can get. Meditation increases the brain's ability to function better.   The improvements are not just temporary ~ they have long-lasting effects.

There are a host of neurological benefits to the brain from meditating. Whereas before it was once thought that only a region or two of the brain was positively impacted, new studies are beginning to show many areas of the brain & body are positively affected. You can read more here. [7]

CHAPTER 4: The Spiritual Benefits of Meditation

What are the Spiritual Benefits of Meditating?

We have learned that there are benefits related to our brain health & our physical health, but there are also many spiritual benefits too:

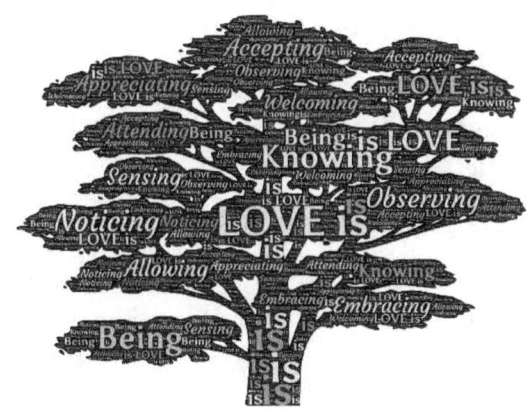

- Helps you reconnect with your inner self
- When connected with self, your dreams come to fruition
- Provides clarity of mind
- Promotes high performance under duress

- Helps develop and foster gratitude. When we are in gratitude more situations to be grateful for come our way

- Long lasting after effects

- You can reap the rewards of having a feeling of connectedness rather than always thinking of self. When we feel connected, we work better as a team. Working better as a team equals more success, more focus & more results

- Decrease in anxious thoughts and feelings as well as mild depression

- Reap the rewards of the body brain connection. If you are healthier, you are more productive

- Meditation can help you set and achieve goals

- Meditation can foster healthier relationships. If you are healthy and happy and at peace, then that state will radiate to those around you

- Increases focus

- Increases creativity

- Increases motivation

CHAPTER 5: Types of Meditation & Meditation Techniques

Although there are many different types of meditation that we can practice, here are 13 to consider...

Centring and Mindfulness
Grounding and Focused
Focusing on Breath
Protective Shielding & Visualisation
Movement Meditation (yoga, tai chi & walking)
Mantra Meditation
Spiritual Meditation
Transcendental Meditation
Loving Kindness Meditation (Metta Meditation)
Guided Meditation
Vipassana Meditation
Chakra Meditation
Labyrinth Meditation

Centring and Mindfulness

Simply put, centring means to return to your inner home being base. During your day how many times do you find yourself thinking about so many different things? These thoughts can lead you on a merry dance all over the place continuously distracting you!

With so many activities and responsibilities to take care of, it's easy to get caught up in the daily mindset of having a busy mind. Centring will help to gently and easily guide you back to your central foundation.

With mindful meditation you learn to pay attention to these random thoughts being fully present as they come in and out of your mind. You are not judging them or engaging with them, you simply observe them and begin to realise the patterns of the mind.

This is a powerful practice as it combines concentration with self-awareness of your bodily sensations, thoughts and feelings. With the focus on your breathing you can catch yourself and choose not to follow these thoughts that do not support or serve you.

This practice of gently brings your thoughts back and centring to the present moment of awareness. Being aware of where we are and what we're doing, and not being overly reactive to what's going on around you.

You will begin to train your mind not to think upon anything else other than what's in the present moment and ultimately feelings of inner peace.

Being mindful means this meditation can be done anywhere. Some people prefer to sit in a quiet place, close their eyes, and focus on their breathing. But you can choose to be mindful at any point of the day, including while you're commuting to work or doing chores.

When practicing mindfulness meditation, you observe your thoughts and emotions but let them pass without judgement.

Technique:
In this meditation, just concentrate on your awareness of the present moment. Start with a single central point, such as your breath, and then expand to include your thoughts, emotions, & sensations.

Find a quiet place with few distractions. Sit in a chair or on the floor. Be comfortable & don't fidget.

Become aware of your breathing and focus on the sensation of air moving in and out of your body as you breathe. Feel your belly rise and fall and the air enters your nostrils and exits your mouth.

Watch every thought come and go. When thoughts come up, don't pay them any attention. Simply note them and return to concentrating on your breathing.

As you finish, sit quietly for a couple of minutes, to re-adjust to & be aware of, where you are.   Get up slowly & drink a glass of water.

Grounding and Focused Meditation

Grounding is similar to rooting yourself, you ground yourself when you connect to the energy of the earth. It involves using any of your five senses.

Walking barefoot in the grass, paddling on the sea shore or standing outside while your bare feet connect with the earth is a great way to ground yourself, taking you out of your head and constant mind chatter into present time awareness.

Nature has a way of healing us and when we consciously connect with it, it's a beautiful sense of returning home. While it's not always possible to get out barefoot in the grass or dig your bare feet into the mud or ocean you can always use your imagination, also known as visualisation.

Technique:
You can start by getting as comfortable as you can. You could sit on a blanket or pillow on the floor, you could lie on your back on the bed or you could stand up & imagine your feet grounding into the earth.

Imagine you are standing tall in a forest deep in the woods somewhere. Begin to breathe in slowly on a count to five.

You could visualise breathing in new energy as to prepare to release stagnant old energy. As you visualise yourself connecting the soles of your feet to the grounds and roots of the earth, begin to imagine filling up those roots with pure light energy.

The next step is to breathe out and release all the old stagnant energy. The point is to visualize as you meditate on what you want.   If you want to release limiting fears and beliefs, then you need to visualise new life entering your body as you release all the stagnant thoughts.

Focusing on Breath

We've talked before about the need to focus on breathing, but there is more to this simple state than meets the eye. Focusing on breath resets your sense of self. It brings you back to centre, and helps you to focus on the simple act of breathing in and out so that you can practice mindfulness. Taking deep breaths consciously brings a true sense of calm & is a good way to alleviate stress. Let the anxiety of the mind go as you rest yourself.

When you focus on breath, you focus on where you are at in the present moment. Present moment practices allow you to quiet and calm your mind. This practice is a very simple achievable process to do anytime, anywhere.

Technique:
As you breathe in through your nose and out through your mouth, concentrate on all the good things you

want to create. Picture white light entering your body and resetting your life force. As you breathe out, picture all the negativity leaving your body and making way for the next light breath.

Protective Shielding & Visualisation

As part of the meditation routine, you can adopt a way to incorporate protective shielding into your life. Shielding is simply another form of visualisation but with shielding you are protecting your own self from negative energies.

Some people are more sensitive than others. When this happens, it's easy to take on the energies of other people. It's easy for other people to say to toughen up or not be so sensitive, but unless you are an empath, you might not understand quite how difficult this is.

Technique:
Practice imagining a shield of protection surrounding you. If you are the claustrophobic type, then picture a shield in front of you rather than something encasing. Use what works best for you. As you meditate on this vision, you will begin to feel more comfortable in places where you are not usually comfortable.

Imagine yourself entering a meeting or a party where you don't know or necessarily feel totally comfortable with people there. This could be the perfect time to practice shielding. Preparation before you go the party or meeting will help support you deal with this type of life scenario.

Visualisation is a great tool which involves the creation of real or unreal images in the mind's eye. You can refer to visual images, images of sound, movement, touch, taste and smell. It is using your imagination to create your will. Bring into your mind's eye all that you desire and want. This is a traditional mind-body technique which can, in turn, help bring about physiological changes in the body and psychological changes in the mind.

Visualising along with deep breathing and affirmations is a powerful trio.

Movement Meditation

Movement meditation is an active form of meditation where the movement will guide you and allow you to find peace in action and focus. Many people are attracted to yoga, tai chi, qigong, gardening, walking in nature and other gentle forms of movement.

Yoga concentrates on breathing, movement, and posture to still your mind, help you relax & control stress.

The practice of yoga dates back to ancient India & possibly much earlier. There are a wide variety of classes and styles of yoga, but they all involve performing a series of postures and controlled breathing exercises which promote flexibility and calm the mind.

The poses require balance and concentration and practitioners are encouraged to focus less on distractions and stay more in the moment.

Whichever style of meditation you decide to try depends on a number of factors. If you have a health condition and are new to yoga, speak to your doctor about which style may be right for you.

Tai chi combines slow, gentle movements, and deep breathing.

In a walking meditation you slow down your pace so that you can focus on each step and the movement of your legs and feet.

Basic house cleaning can be a movement meditation by allowing the gentle movements to guide you, your mind is free to wander and explore within itself.

Mantra Meditation

A mantra is a syllable, word, or phrase that is repeated during meditation. Mantras can be spoken, chanted, whispered, or repeated in the mind. Most mantra meditation techniques have two essential components: mindfulness meditation and mantra recitation or chanting.

This type of meditation uses a repetitive sound to clear the mind and focus on a word, phrase or sound such as the "OM", this method is prominent in many doctrines including Hindu and Buddhist teachings. The mantra can be spoken loudly or quietly.

After chanting the mantra for a while, it will allow you to be more alert and in tune with your environment, and experience deeper levels of awareness. Some people prefer mantra meditation as they find it easier to focus on a word than on their breath. This is a good practice for those who don't find silence easy and can enjoy the repetition.

Technique:
Here are a couple of examples:

Allow yourself some private time & space & repeat Nam Myoho Renge Kyo [naam my oh ho ren gay key o] as often as possible. This can be done while sitting alone or while walking the dog!

It is said to chant Nam Myoho Renge Kyo is to bring forth the pure and fundamental energy of life, honouring the dignity and possibility of our ordinary lives. You can read more in the references section [8]

If you have trouble sleeping you can try the Shring mantra. Use a prayer bead necklace or Mala that has 108 beads. The mala is used so that one can focus on the meaning or sound of the mantra rather than counting its repetitions. One repetition is usually said for each bead while turning the thumb clockwise around each bead. When arriving at the Guru bead, some say that Hindus and Tibetan Buddhists traditionally turn the mala around and then go back in the opposite direction. However, some teachers in the Tibetan tradition say that this is superstitious and therefore not important.   You can read more below [9]

Repeating 'shring' 'shring' 'shring' repeatedly definitely sends me to sleep!

Spiritual Meditation

At its core, spiritual meditation is the mindful practice of connection to something that is greater, vaster, and deeper than the individual self.

Spiritual meditation is used in the Christian faith and eastern religions such as Hinduism and Daoism.   It is similar to prayer in that you reflect on the silence around you and seek a deeper connection with your God or the Divine Universe.

Spiritual meditation and contemplation can be practiced at home or in a place of worship, this practice is of benefit for those who thrive in silence and seek spiritual growth.

Essential oils are commonly used to evoke and heighten the experience these include:

Frankincense
Myrrh

Sage
Cedar
Sandalwood
Palo Santo

Transcendental

Transcendental meditation was reportedly founded
by Maharishi Mahesh Yogi. Transcendental
meditation is the most studied type by scientists & is
typically a Sanskrit sound learned from a
Transcendental Meditation teacher.

Transcendental meditation is slightly more organized
and structured than Mantra meditation, with each
student receiving a specific mantra based on a
number of different factors such as birth year and
sometimes gender. This mantra is repeated along
with the focus on your breath. This practice is
believed to be the most popular type of meditation
around the world.

Loving Kindness Meditation (Metta Meditation)

Metta meditation, also called Loving Kindness
Meditation, is the practice of directing well wishes
toward others. Those who practice recite specific
words and phrases meant to evoke warm-hearted
feelings. This is also commonly found in mindfulness
and vipassana meditation.

Technique:
It's typically practiced while sitting in a comfortable, relaxed position. After a few deep breaths, you repeat the following words slowly and steadily. "May I be happy. May I be well. May I be safe. May I be peaceful and at ease."

After a period of directing this loving kindness toward yourself, you may begin to picture a family member or friend who has helped you and repeat the mantra again, this time replacing "I" with "you."

As you continue the meditation, you can bring other members of your family, friends, neighbours, or people in your life to mind. Practitioners are also encouraged to visualize people they have difficulty with.

Finally, you end the meditation with the universal mantra: "May all being everywhere be happy."

Guided Meditation

Guided meditation, which is sometimes also called guided imagery or visualisation, is a method of meditation in which you form mental pictures or situations that you find relaxing.

This process is typically led by a guide or teacher, hence "guided." It's often suggested to use as many senses as possible, such as smell, sounds, and textures, to evoke calmness in your relaxing space.

Vipassana Meditation

Vipassana meditation is an ancient Indian form of meditation & is the oldest of Buddhist meditation practices. It means to see things as they really are. It was taught in India more than 2,500 years ago. The mindfulness meditation movement in the United States has its roots in this tradition.

The goal of vipassana meditation is self-transformation through self-observation. Vipassana or insight meditation is a clear awareness of exactly what is happening as it happens.

This is accomplished through disciplined attention to physical sensations in the body, to establish a deep connection between the mind and body. The continuous interconnectedness results in a balanced mind full of love and compassion.

We to pay attention to the changes taking place in all our experiences large or small through our senses. We learn to listen to our own thoughts without being caught up in them.

The object of Vipassana meditation practice is to learn to see the truth of impermanence. Vipassana, in this tradition, is typically taught during a 10 day course, and students are expected to follow a set of rules throughout the entirety of the time, including abstaining from all intoxicants, telling lies, stealing, sexual activity, and killing any species.

Chakra Meditation

Chakra is an ancient Sanskrit word which translates to "wheel". Chakras refer to the centres of energy and spiritual power in the body. There are thought to be seven chakras. Each chakra is located at a different part of the body and each has a corresponding colour. The chakras are considered to be wheel-like energy centres that are not physically discernible but belong to the subtle spiritual body and connect it to the material one. The 7 main chakras are situated along the spine from the sacrum at the bottom up to the crown at the top of the head.

Chakra meditation is made up of relaxation techniques focused on bringing balance and well-being to each of the chakras. Some of these techniques include visually picturing each chakra in the body and its corresponding colour. Some people may choose to light incense or use crystals, colour coded for each chakra to help them concentrate during the meditation.

The Root Chakra
The root chakra, or Muladhara in Sanskrit, is located at the base of the spine. It governs the way we connect to the outside world and oversees our basic needs for stability, food and shelter. It is associated with the colour red and the earth element.

The Sacral Chakra
Svadhisthana, the sacral chakra, is located below the

navel. This chakra is intimately linked to our sexuality and creative process. Its energy encourages us to explore the world and use our creativity to find artistic outlets and adapt to change. Its base colour is orange and its element is water.

The Solar Plexus Chakra
The Sanskrit name Manipura means City of Jewels. This chakra is located between the rib cage and the navel. It is believed to be a source of personal agency and self-esteem in that it translates our desires into action. Physically, it helps regulate digestion. Its colour is yellow and it is associated with the fire element.

The Heart Chakra
Anahata, the heart chakra, means "unstuck" in Sanskrit. This chakra lies at the middle of your cardiovascular system and is connected to organs such as the heart and lungs. The heart chakra is associated with a person's emotional profile, such as their natural generosity and ability to appreciate compassion and connectedness. Its colour is green and its element is air.

The Throat Chakra
Vishuddha, the throat chakra, governs the neck, mouth, tongue and other physical elements of the throat area. It regulates how we communicate and allows us to express ourselves skilfully. Confidence and understanding are related to this chakra. Its colour is blue and its element is ether.

The Third Eye Chakra
Ajna is located behind the forehead, at the level of the space between the eyebrows. The "third eye" chakra governs intuition and insight, especially at spiritual levels. A receptive and balanced ajna chakra empowers us to notice interconnections that exist in this world and beyond. Its colour is indigo and its element is light.

The Crown Chakra
Sahasrara, the crown chakra, is situated at the top of the head. Also known as the "thousand petal lotus" chakra, it is considered to be the most spiritual of the core chakras as it governs spiritual consciousness and the potential for awakening to the dimension of the divine. Its colour is purple (or white) and it embodies the spirit.

Labyrinth Meditation

A labyrinth is an ancient symbol that relates to wholeness.   It combines the imagery of the circle and the spiral into a meandering but purposeful path. The Labyrinth represents a journey to our own centre and back again out into the world. Labyrinths have long been used as meditation and prayer tools. We can walk it. It is a metaphor for life's journey. It is a symbol that creates a sacred space and place and takes us out of our ego to "That Which Is Within."

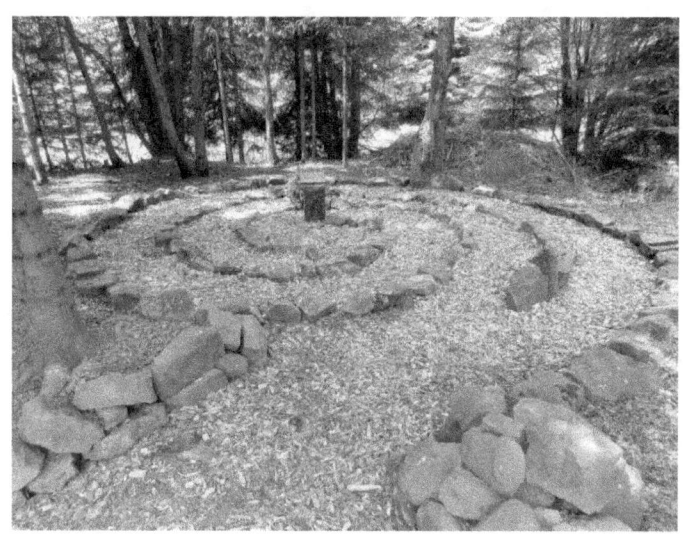

Technique:
Stand in front of the entrance to the labyrinth. ...
Centre yourself by taking a couple of deep breaths. ...
Acknowledge your coming meditative or spiritual journey within the labyrinth. ...
Begin your walk. ...
Continue to walk. ...
Pause on reaching the centre. ...
Walk out.

As you can see, meditation has a multitude of benefits. These benefits make their way into your mind, body, and spirit. Not only do you reap the rewards and benefits of incorporating meditation into your daily life, so does everyone else around you.

Meditation is not difficult to learn and it is not difficult to keep up the pace. Some days it will feel easy and sometimes difficult, the trick to stay with it, no matter how it feels. In only 10 minutes a day, you could be on your way to a brand new you.

CHAPTER 6: Making Time not Excuses

Resolve to make time for yourself instead of inventing reasons why you can't

The biggest reason or excuse people say that they haven't tried meditation is because they say they don't have enough time. Not having enough time is not a valid excuse. We can all find 10 minutes in a day where we do little or nothing

You would find time to go to a physiotherapist if you had an injury & you would make time to go to a doctor if became ill. So instead of waiting until stress & anxiety produce physical symptoms in your body, be kind to yourself & find a few minutes to recharge your batteries & work your way toward a whole and complete life.

You could take 10 minutes out of your lunch hour or set your alarm 10 minutes earlier three times per week or go to bed 10 minutes later.

Depending on your personality you could vary these times so it doesn't feel repetitive or you could set an alarm on your smart phone at a set time each day.

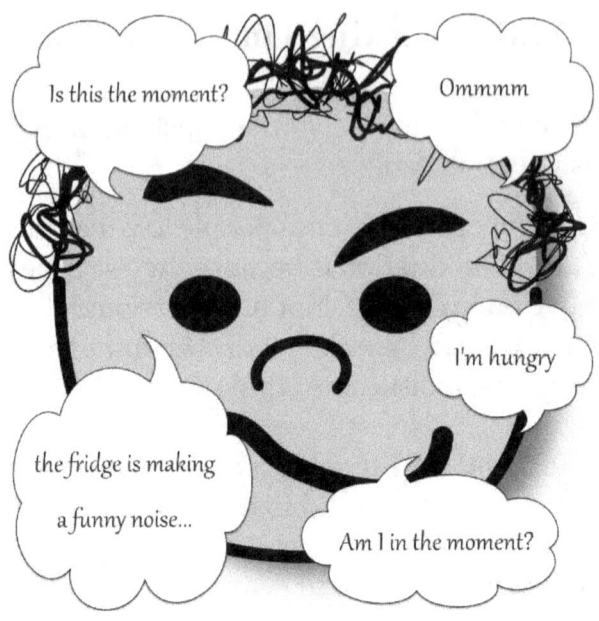

Mini Meditation Sessions - How to Perform Them Anywhere

You can meditate just about anywhere. You don't need to have a meditation session deep in the woods or sit in a special corner of your room wearing long flowing robes or light candles.

If you're waiting in a queue or a long line, you can practice deep breathing. If you are sitting in a waiting room, on a bus or a train; just drift off into your own world & visualize something much better for yourself than standing in line waiting for stamps at the post office.

You can alleviate the stress out of waiting too ~ visualise, centre, ground, & take deep breaths. You could use the shielding technique as mentioned in Chapter 5.

You can meditate anywhere at any time where it is safe to do so [obviously not whilst driving the car!]

CHAPTER 7: Awareness of Self

What does that mean?   If you feel you are going into a negative spiral, being out of kilter it's important to check in with yourself. You can take control of your mind ~ you don't need it to control you.

Here are a few ways to check in with yourself when you feel life is getting way too busy & your mind is racing:

- Focus on gratitude to increase happiness which, in turn, will increase positive thoughts & then productivity. Just write down 5 things you are grateful for today. It could be something as simple as "I'm grateful that the car started" or "I'm grateful for central heating" or "I'm grateful for a roof over my head".

- Sit quietly & meditate for a few minutes. Allow thoughts to pass through without making them 'wrong'. Just being mindful of them is a great way to check in with yourself. When you allow the thoughts to come, you can consciously practice letting them go easily.   Many turn to medication as the answer, but for those seeking alternative benefits without medication, meditation is a healthier choice.

- Sticking with it when your mind wants to fight against meditation is also a great way to check in with yourself. When you get frustrated & irritated with meditation, [it happens!] you can make a new commitment to it. Maybe get a trusted friend or meditation buddy who will hold you accountable & practice of meditation with you.

- Sticking with it when it all seems too much. Check in & find out what is really the problem -. Don't quit & don't give up. Keep going.

- Check in & monitor your thoughts – Is the thing you are worried about happening exactly at this moment? If not, try 'present moment' practice together with meditative breathing.

- Recreate & restructure your thoughts – could you turn that negative emotion into something else? For example, could you be grateful for something good rather than focusing on something not working for you? You could practice meditating on this.

- Being aware of yourself, visualisation & meditation work hand in hand together – remember you can meditate with deep breathing while you visualise your way to happiness and peace and calm.

CHAPTER 8: How to Get Started & Step-by-Step Guide

How to Get Started in a Few Minutes a Day

Everything can be a meditation if you give it your full awareness & build it into your life as a habit. It is going to become your new regime, just like waking up, brushing your teeth & having a shower.

There is always a learning curve whenever you take on something new. This doesn't take a lot of time but it does require you doing a bit each & every day until it becomes a new habit.

One day you will get to a point where you could not imagine meditation not being a part of your daily life. You will wonder how you got along without it...

Meditation techniques:

As discussed in Chapter 5, it's important to familiarise yourself with the various mindfulness techniques & choose the ones which are best for you. Choose the ones which are in perfect alignment with your thoughts & lifestyle.

You might want to incorporate your new-found breathing techniques with your ability to shield; or you might find that visualization with centring works best for you.

Whichever combination you choose, just make sure it works for you, your life and your particular situation. You will be able to mix and match these techniques according to the scenario in which is presenting itself. For example, if you are feeling stressed about a new job, perhaps breathing and visualization will work best.

However, if you find you are nervous about going into a social setting where you will know no one, perhaps using the shielding and grounding techniques will work best for you.

How to Begin:

Any new endeavour takes time to get used to. Just like anything else, you don't want to jump in too much too soon. If you are exercising for the first time, you certainly wouldn't run a 5K on the first day. Here are a few tips to get you started:

- Start slowly – no matter how excited you are about beginning your meditation journey, it's important to start slow. You don't want to get overzealous and fall short. Often when people start something new, they go all out and get overwhelmed & feel burned out. They have good intentions, but they don't always stick with it. Meditation can be overwhelming in the beginning until you learn how to train your brain and guide yourself back to centre.

- Set up a space – It's important to set up a space that you can call your own. It does not have to be anything elaborate. It just needs to be somewhere meaningful to you. It could be a corner of your sitting room or in front of the window of your bedroom on the floor. Wherever it is, make it your own.

- Create a routine – it's important, just as you would with any new endeavour, to create a routine. Just stick to the time you choose & keep to your routine.

- Stand in integrity, and do what you say you will, when you say you will – if you say you are going to practice meditation, then take it on whole heartedly. Set an example for the rest of your family and show them what it looks like to be a role model in integrity.

- Maybe you would find it easier to get a partner - & not go it alone – meditation can be fun when you partner with other people. Find an accountability partner or someone to join in the fun with you.

- Let everyone know you are taking on this practice whether they want to join you or agree with you, or not. Be up front and clear that meditation is important to you and you fully intend to reap the benefits. They will reap the rewards as well when they see a brand new you.

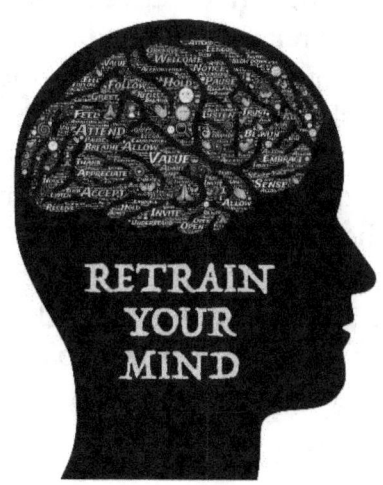

Step-by-Step Guide

1] Find somewhere peaceful & quiet, sit comfortably in a chair, with your feet on ground. Have your hands relaxed in lap do not cross your legs. Keep your back straight but relaxed.

2] Start with eyes open and take some deep breaths, lungs feel up and let breath go to normal, observe body, feet on floor body relaxing, notice sounds and how the breath in the body feels can feel it stomach, chest or diaphragm, just notice rise and fall sensation of the body as you breathe normally through the nose and out of mouth, notice sounds around you, as you follow that movement of breathe the mind will wander away, just acknowledge and come back to that rising and fall of breath, this is normal. Lots of thoughts are perfectly normal.

3] Just acknowledge that you've taken time for the mind and body to relax. The mind is always changing, just allow the process to unfold you are learning a new skill.

4] Allow the sounds around you to come and go and noticing the mind, then the movement of the breath in the body, just notice the breath, notice as the mind wanders and gently coming back to the breath again, the mind does wander bring back to breath then the attention to your body, and the sounds around.

5]   Notice how you feel, this exercise is about being at ease with the mind as it is.

6]   Meditation isn't about stopping your thoughts just allow them to pass by observing them & letting them go.

7]   A skill just takes regular practice to improve. Set aside 10 minutes a day, you will start to feel comfortable with you own mind. Research has proven that even 2 minutes per day for 21 days is more beneficial than 10 mins once a week.   It appears regular repetition reaps greater benefits.

Other ways to get started:
- join a yoga class, personally I recommend Iyengar yoga as the teaching is very precise
- join a tai chi class
- go for a walk & think only of your steps & legs & feet ~ find a lovely space like a park, or woodland or beside the sea

Chapter 9: History of Meditation

The practice of meditation is of prehistoric origin, and is found throughout history, especially in religious context, archaeologists and scholars agree that it's been around for about 5,000 years.

The earliest documented evidence of meditation stems from the Hindu teachings of Veda in ancient India from around 1,500 BCE (Before Common Era) The practice of Chinese Taoist and Indian Buddhism was practiced 600-500 BCE.

The Silk Road was an ancient network of trade routes that connected the East and West. It was central to cultural interaction between the regions for many centuries, & it was via this route that meditation was introduced to other oriental countries.

Between 400- 100 BCE The Yoga Sutras of Patanjali were compiled on the theory and practice of Yoga being the most translated ancient Indian text in the medieval era.

Between 400 BCE and 200 CE (Common Era) The Bhagavad Gita was written; a very popular scripture and epic poem that discusses the philosophy of yoga, meditation and how to live a spiritual life.

In 653 CE with the growth of Japanese Buddhism from the 8th century onwards, meditative practices were brought to, and further developed in, Japan. This is where the first meditation hall is known to have opened.

Moving forward to the 18th Century, translations of the ancient scriptures began to travel with scholars to the West.

Meditation and the spiritual journey of self-discovery was popularised by Hermann Hesse when in 1922 he published *Siddhartha* A philosophical fiction of the Buddha's spiritual journey.

It was in 1927 when *The Tibetan Book of Dead* by Dr. Walter Y. Evans-Wentz was published, that westerners were attracted to Tibetan Buddhism. When Timothy Leary commented in 1964 "that this book is a key to the innermost recesses of the human mind, and a guide for initiates, and for those who are seeking the spiritual path of liberation", many became interested.

The Vipassanā movement, also called the Insight Meditation Movement, refers to a branch of modern Burmese Buddhism which gained widespread popularity from the 1950s. Its western derivatives have been popularised since the 1970s, and gave rise to the mindfulness movement.

The American Beat author Jack Kerouac wrote *The Dharma Bums*. The protagonist's search for a "Buddhist" context to his experiences. The book had a significant influence on the Hippie counterculture of the 1960s. In 1968 the English rock band, the Beatles, travelled to Northern India to the Ashram & School of Maharishi Mahesh Yogi to learn Transcendental Meditation. This received worldwide media coverage and changed Western attitudes about Indian spirituality and encouraged the study of Transcendental Meditation.

During the 60s & 70s Hatha yoga and Transcendental meditation began to gain popularity in Europe and America as more and more people testify about the benefits of a regular practice.

It was in 1979 Jon Kabat-Zinn, an American professor emeritus of medicine and the creator of the Stress Reduction Clinic and the Centre for Mindfulness in Medicine, Health Care, and Society at the University of Massachusetts Medical School began to treat patients with chronic illnesses which gained the interest of mindfulness practices and meditation in the medical and scientific world.

In 1997 Eckhart Tolle published *The Power of Now: A Guide to Spiritual Enlightenment* and introduced the reader to present-moment awareness and how to tune into themselves. This was described as a re-working of "Buddhism mixed with mysticism and a few references to Jesus Christ, a sort of New Age re-working of Zen".

In 2003 Dr. Deepak Chopra, an Indian American, popularised Meditation through his book *The Spontaneous Fulfilment of Desire*, writing about the awareness of the awesome powers within us. Through specific meditative principles and exercises he provides the tools with which to create a positive and fulfilling life.

Fast forward to now where the internet has opened up so much to all of us to explore, discover and learn. There are many Teachers, Gurus, Masters and Facilitators offering every type of Meditation giving a different spin in a secular world. The internet has made it accessible for everybody, who has a slight interest in finding out more, to try.

Fundamentally Meditation offers you a way back to peace and stillness in our busy lives and schedules. You can find Meditation classes at many health clubs, fitness schools, meetups, spiritual retreats, medical clinics, and wellness centres and many different types of meditation classes.

However, if you are a complete novice with not much time or resources to go out to a class, you can start with as little as 10 minutes a day in your own home. Using our simple techniques, which we share with you here, we really can support you in many areas and aspects of your life. When you **train the mind for a happier, healthy existence, and** focus totally, you can create a successful life for yourself.

Let me know if you would like a FREE 10 minute Meditation mp3…

Whatever you choose make sure you enjoy every single moment. We wish you every success!

About the Authors

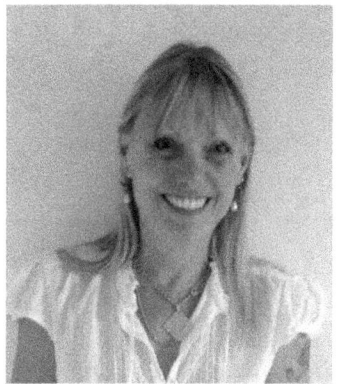

Hello, my name is Susie Ellis, mother of four, a qualified hypnotherapist & business & lifestyle coach.

I started my working life as a PA for a commercial Estate Agent in Green Park, London & then when I later moved to Norfolk, I became PA to the Finance Director of a Blue-Chip Company. The first gave me hands on experience in a start-up & the second a fantastic grounding in the 'bottom line'. During a management buy-out, another fantastic learning curve, I found myself being eased sideways so I left & started up my own business as a consultant.

My first project was to overhaul all the working processes & systems for a company specialising in laying oil pipelines in Russia! It was a fixed 6 month contract & I then had to employ staff to take over the running of the company. Since then I have specialised in troubleshooting.

In 2010 I qualified as a hypnotherapist & I now use those skills, including NLP, in my coaching business. I find that mindset & self-esteem are as important to a business as financial reporting.

We specialise in helping people and businesses excel in all that they do. We can help you achieve...providing accountability, guidance, systems & ideas...see www.susieellis.net

Also, over the years I have become more & more interested in maintaining a healthy lifestyle, eating organic & unprocessed food & avoiding pharmaceuticals. I have developed a lifelong interest in food & it's effect on our health which began when one of my children was cured of 'hyperactivity syndrome' by cutting out food additives & colourings from his diet...see www.susieellis.org

Then I progressed to researching the ingredients in the personal care products & makeup we were using. I was horrified to read about SLS & Propylene glycol for a start! Let alone what else I uncovered during the process. I was encouraged to learn the truth, help others, & share my findings & ideas with the world...see www.behindthetruth.co.uk

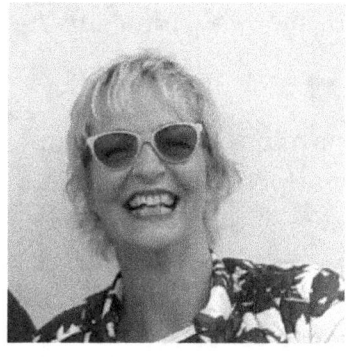

Hello, my name is Louisa Marsh [also known as Karuna Louisa]

I'm a Clarity Coach & Vision Board Workshop facilitator supporting you to uncover and live from your Heart's Desire, to Empower you to make healthy choices to live a life of Joy, Abundance & Prosperity.

I am Brighton based (UK) and universally available via Skype or Zoom

I am a great fan of entrepreneurship & supporting people to discover their Personal Power and Passion, I work with the principles of The Law of Attraction

I am a mother of two & have a big Yes & passion for life!

I lived in a community for four years where our shared goals were self-awareness, personal development and celebration. I learned to share myself from a place of love, authenticity, integrity and creative self-expression.

I have been a meditator and for many years, and am qualified to teach many different practices both silent and dynamic.

I am an excellent facilitator and have a natural ability to tune in to the needs and deeper processes of people, supporting you from my heart. I have a finely tuned intuition and bring my presence and love.

I can work with you on a one to one basis to help you find what holds you back from having the life you truly love and choose.

I also run workshops and retreats and offer Vision Board days, Meditation & one to one coaching using The Law of Attraction

Credits & References

1   Chapter 3/1 ~
       www.nyaspubs.onlinelibrary.wiley.com/doi/a
       bs/10.1111/nyas.12348

2   Chapter 3/7

       www.ncbi.nlm.nih.gov/pmc/articles/PMC432
       5657/

3   Chapter 3/10 Text attribution
       www.sciencedirect.com/science/article/pii/S
       1871187106000289

4   Chapter 3/20
       www.forbes.com/sites/jeenacho/2016/03/05
       /increase-happiness-and-sense-of-well-being-
       through-meditation/#3d190d5e2adb

5   Chapter 3/22
       www.journals.plos.org/plosone/article?id=10.
       1371/journal.pone.0062817

6   Chapter 3/22
       www.theguardian.com/science/blog/2016/m
       ar/03/could-meditation-really-help-slow-the-
       ageing-process

7   Chapter 3/23
     www.researchgate.net/publication/273774412
     _The_neuroscience_of_mindfulness_meditatio
     n

8   Chapter 5
     www.sgi.org/about-us/buddhist-
     concepts/the-meaning-of-nam-myoho-renge-
     kyo.html

9   Chapter 5
     www.en.wikipedia.org/wiki/Buddhist_prayer
     _beads

Labyrinth image by Kascha Pixabay
Brain & other word cloud images by John Hain
Pixabay

Contact us:

We are more than happy to answer questions & hear your experiences

so do get in touch...

karuna@karunalouisamarsh.com

info@susieellis.net

Louisa
facebook.com/louisa.marsh7
twitter @karunalouisa1
instagram.com/karunalouisa

Susie
facebook.com/susieellis.inc
twitter @_Susie Ellis
instagram.com/trulyspecial

Journal

This is where you can record your thoughts every week for a year

You can keep a note of the highs & lows in your meditation journey & see where it leads you

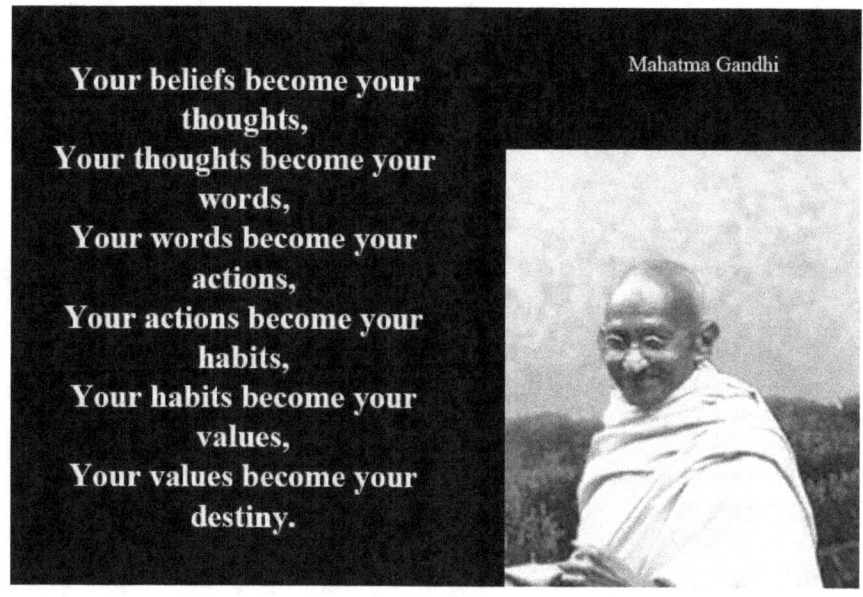

Your beliefs become your thoughts,
Your thoughts become your words,
Your words become your actions,
Your actions become your habits,
Your habits become your values,
Your values become your destiny.

Mahatma Gandhi

Week 1

....
....
....
....
....
....
....
....
....
....
....
....
....
....
....
....
....
....
....
....
....
....
....
....
....
....
....
....
....
....
....
....
....

Week 2

··

··

··

··

··

··

··

··

··

··

··

··

··

··

··

··

··

··

··

··

··

··

··

··

··

··

··

··

··

··

Week 3

....
....
....
....
....
....
....
....
....
....
....
....
....
....
....
....
....
....
....
....
....
....
....
....
....
....
....
....
....
....

Week 4

....
....
....
....
....
....
....
....
....
....
....
....
....
....
....
....
....
....
....
....
....
....
....
....
....
....
....
....
....
....
....
....

Week 5

....
....
....
....
....
....
....
....
....
....
....
....
....
....
....
....
....
....
....
....
....
....
....
....
....
....
....
....
....
....
....

Week 6

....
....
....
....
....
....
....
....
....
....
....
....
....
....
....
....
....
....
....
....
....
....
....
....
....
....
....
....
....
....
....
....

Week 7

....
....
....
....
....
....
....
....
....
....
....
....
....
....
....
....
....
....
....
....
....
....
....
....
....
....
....
....
....
....

Week 8

....
....
....
....
....
....
....
....
....
....
....
....
....
....
....
....
....
....
....
....
....
....
....
....
....
....
....
....
....
....

Week 9

....
....
....
....
....
....
....
....
....
....
....
....
....
....
....
....
....
....
....
....
....
....
....
....
....
....
....
....
....
....
....

Week 10

....
....
....
....
....
....
....
....
....
....
....
....
....
....
....
....
....
....
....
....
....
....
....
....
....
....
....
....
....
....
....
....

Week 11

Week 12

....

....

....

....

....

....

....

....

....

....

....

....

....

....

....

....

....

....

....

....

....

....

....

....

....

....

....

....

....

....

....

Week 13

....
....
....
....
....
....
....
....
....
....
....
....
....
....
....
....
....
....
....
....
....
....
....
....
....
....
....
....
....
....
....

Week 14

....
....
....
....
....
....
....
....
....
....
....
....
....
....
....
....
....
....
....
....
....
....
....
....
....
....
....
....
....
....
....

Week 15

....
....
....
....
....
....
....
....
....
....
....
....
....
....
....
....
....
....
....
....
....
....
....
....
....
....
....
....
....
....

Week 16

Week 17

Week 18

....
....
....
....
....
....
....
....
....
....
....
....
....
....
....
....
....
....
....
....
....
....
....
....
....
....
....
....
....
....
....
....

Week 19

Week 20

....
....
....
....
....
....
....
....
....
....
....
....
....
....
....
....
....
....
....
....
....
....
....
....
....
....
....
....
....
....

Week 21

....
....
....
....
....
....
....
....
....
....
....
....
....
....
....
....
....
....
....
....
....
....
....
....
....
....
....
....
....
....
....

Week 22

Week 23

....
....
....
....
....
....
....
....
....
....
....
....
....
....
....
....
....
....
....
....
....
....
....
....
....
....
....
....
....
....
....
....

Week 24

....
....
....
....
....
....
....
....
....
....
....
....
....
....
....
....
....
....
....
....
....
....
....
....
....
....
....
....
....
....

Week 25

Week 26

....

....

....

....

....

....

....

....

....

....

....

....

....

....

....

....

....

....

....

....

....

....

....

....

....

....

....

....

....

....

....

....

....

Week 27

....
....
....
....
....
....
....
....
....
....
....
....
....
....
....
....
....
....
....
....
....
....
....
....
....
....
....
....
....
....
....

Week 28

....
....
....
....
....
....
....
....
....
....
....
....
....
....
....
....
....
....
....
....
....
....
....
....
....
....
....
....
....
....
....

Week 29

....
....
....
....
....
....
....
....
....
....
....
....
....
....
....
....
....
....
....
....
....
....
....
....
....
....
....
....
....
....
....
....

Week 30

....
....
....
....
....
....
....
....
....
....
....
....
....
....
....
....
....
....
....
....
....
....
....
....
....
....
....
....
....
....
....
....

Week 31

....
....
....
....
....
....
....
....
....
....
....
....
....
....
....
....
....
....
....
....
....
....
....
....
....
....
....
....
....
....
....
....

Week 32

....
....
....
....
....
....
....
....
....
....
....
....
....
....
....
....
....
....
....
....
....
....
....
....
....
....
....
....
....
....
....
....

Week 33

....
....
....
....
....
....
....
....
....
....
....
....
....
....
....
....
....
....
....
....
....
....
....
....
....
....
....
....
....
....
....
....

Week 34

....
....
....
....
....
....
....
....
....
....
....
....
....
....
....
....
....
....
....
....
....
....
....
....
....
....
....
....
....
....

Week 35

....
....
....
....
....
....
....
....
....
....
....
....
....
....
....
....
....
....
....
....
....
....
....
....
....
....
....
....
....
....
....

Week 36

....
....
....
....
....
....
....
....
....
....
....
....
....
....
....
....
....
....
....
....
....
....
....
....
....
....
....
....
....
....
....

Week 37

....
....
....
....
....
....
....
....
....
....
....
....
....
....
....
....
....
....
....
....
....
....
....
....
....
....
....
....
....
....

Week 38

....
....
....
....
....
....
....
....
....
....
....
....
....
....
....
....
....
....
....
....
....
....
....
....
....
....
....
....
....
....

Week 39

....
....
....
....
....
....
....
....
....
....
....
....
....
....
....
....
....
....
....
....
....
....
....
....
....
....
....
....
....
....

Week 40

....
....
....
....
....
....
....
....
....
....
....
....
....
....
....
....
....
....
....
....
....
....
....
....
....
....
....
....
....
....

Week 41

....
....
....
....
....
....
....
....
....
....
....
....
....
....
....
....
....
....
....
....
....
....
....
....
....
....
....
....
....
....

Week 42

....

....

....

....

....

....

....

....

....

....

....

....

....

....

....

....

....

....

....

....

....

....

....

....

....

....

....

....

....

....

Week 43

....
....
....
....
....
....
....
....
....
....
....
....
....
....
....
....
....
....
....
....
....
....
....
....
....
....
....
....
....
....
....
....
....

Week 44

....
....
....
....
....
....
....
....
....
....
....
....
....
....
....
....
....
....
....
....
....
....
....
....
....
....
....
....
....
....
....
....
....

Week 45

....
....
....
....
....
....
....
....
....
....
....
....
....
....
....
....
....
....
....
....
....
....
....
....
....
....
....
....
....
....
....

Week 46

··
··
··
··
··
··
··
··
··
··
··
··
··
··
··
··
··
··
··
··
··
··
··
··
··
··
··
··
··
··
··

Week 47

....
....
....
....
....
....
....
....
....
....
....
....
....
....
....
....
....
....
....
....
....
....
....
....
....
....
....
....
....
....

Week 48

....
....
....
....
....
....
....
....
....
....
....
....
....
....
....
....
....
....
....
....
....
....
....
....
....
....
....
....
....

Week 49

....
....
....
....
....
....
....
....
....
....
....
....
....
....
....
....
....
....
....
....
....
....
....
....
....
....
....
....
....
....

Week 50

··
··
··
··
··
··
··
··
··
··
··
··
··
··
··
··
··
··
··
··
··
··
··
··
··
··
··
··
··
··
··

Week 51

....
....
....
....
....
....
....
....
....
....
....
....
....
....
....
....
....
....
....
....
....
....
....
....
....
....
....
....
....
....
....

Week 52

....
....
....
....
....
....
....
....
....
....
....
....
....
....
....
....
....
....
....
....
....
....
....
....
....
....
....
....
....
....